Keto Cocktails for Beginners

Learn How to Create your Favorite Keto-Friendly Alcohol Drinks at Home to Lose Weight and Have Fun

Jenny Kern

Table Of Contents

Introduction

Are you eager to know how to make perfect keto cocktails for your family, friends or guests? What ingredients to put in sangria? Which method to choose to prepare Daiquiri? Which alcohol base is best for Mojito? What drinks serve as excellent aperitifs or digestives? This cookbook for both professional bartenders and home cocktail aficionados answers all of the above questions and more. I hope that the cocktails I have to offer you can have fun in their realization and that you will like it. Enjoy.

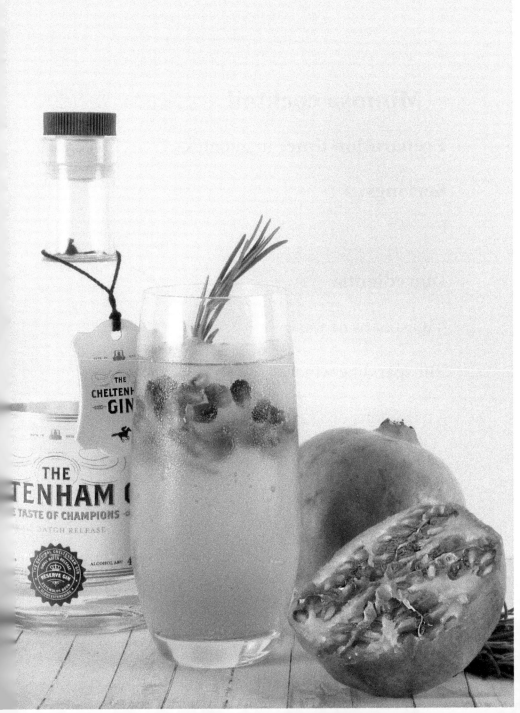

Wine and Champagne Keto Cocktails

Mimosa cocktail

Preparation time: 10 minutes

Servings: 2

Ingredients:

5 teaspoons or 1/2 b

Rut sparkling wine

5 teaspoons or 1/2 orange juice

1slice of orange to garnish

Directions:

To prepare the Mimosa, squeeze the orange - about half - and pour the juice into a flute.

Add the very cold brut sparkling wine

From the remaining orange, make a crescent-shaped slice, slightly cutting the slice so that you can apply it to the glass.

Your Mimosa cocktail is ready to be sipped.

Tips:

Mimosa cocktails should be consumed immediately.

Passion mimosa

Preparation time: 10 minutes

Servings: 2

Ingredients:

4 tablespoons of passion fruit juice

1 tablespoon of triple sec

5oz. of champagne

Strawberry to decorate

Directions:

Pour the passion fruit juice into a champagne flute.

Also, add the triple sec and finally the champagne.

With the bar spoon, mix gently, preventing the release of the bubbles from champagne.

Wash and cut the strawberries in half and use them to decorate the glass.

Alternatively, you can use mimosa sprigs to be fixed on the fluted stem.

Champagne Margaritas

Preparation time: 5 minutes

Servings: 2

Ingredients:

1 bottle champagne

½ cup orange liqueur

1 cup tequila

½ cup fresh lime juice

2 ounces simple syrup

¼ cup fresh mint leaves

Salt, for rim

Lime wedge, for rim

Directions:

Run the lime wedge around the rim of each glass and dip in the salt.

Combine champagne, orange liqueur, tequila, lime juice, mint, and simple syrup in a large pitcher. Mix well.

Pour into glasses and garnish with a lime wedge.

Sicilian Sunset Champagne with Lemon

Preparation time: 10 minutes

Servings: 4

Ingredients:

1 cup Prosecco, which is an Italian sparkling wine

2 cups ice cubes

1 cup cranberry juice

Zest from 2 lemons

1 cup orange juice

Directions:

Add the ice cubes to a pitcher.

Pour the Prosecco wine into the pitcher, along with cranberry and orange juice. Stir the mixture well.

Get champagne flutes. Pour the mixture into them.

Sprinkle with lemon zest, and serve.

Pomegranate Champagne

Preparation time: 10 minutes

Servings: 6

Ingredients:

1 750-ml bottle sparkling wine or champagne

¼ cup brandy

½ cup ginger ale

4 cups ice, crushed

2 cups pomegranate juice

Optional ingredient: pomegranate seeds

Directions:

Mix the wine, brandy, ginger ale, ice, and pomegranate juice in a pitcher.

Pour the mixture into glasses.

Garnish each glass with pomegranate seeds, if using.

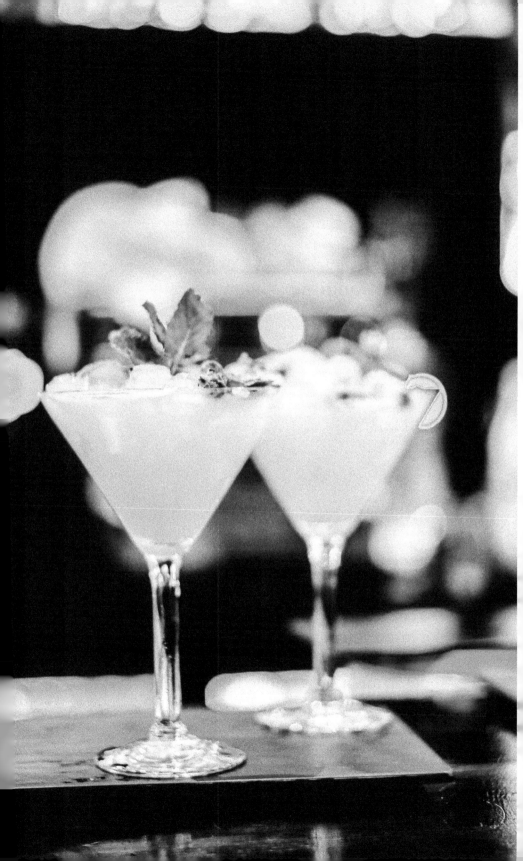

Gin Keto Cocktails

Martini Royale cocktail

Preparation time: 5 minutes

Servings: 1

Ingredients:

Pink Martini

An orange wedge

Martini Prosecco Sigillo Blu

Directions:

Put 1/2 part of Pink Martini and 1/2 part of Prosecco in a hurricane or balloon glass with lots of ice.

Squeeze an orange wedge inside.

Serve for an aperitif or after dinner.

Grapefruit Sangria

Preparation time: 10 minutes

Servings: 7

Ingredients:

½ cup gin or vodka, whichever you prefer

½ cup ruby red grapefruit, cut into four equivalent portions, then cut

½ cup Simple Syrup

½ cup white grapefruit, cut into half-wheels

1 bottle pinot grigio

soda water, as required

Directions:

Mix all of the ingredients apart from the soda water in a big ceramic or glass container.

Place in your fridge, covered, for a minimum of 4 hours (preferably overnight).

Serve over ice and top with soda water.

French 75

Preparation time: 10 minutes

Servings: 2

Ingredients:

8 milliliters sugar syrup

15 milliliters lemon juice

45 milliliters London dry gin

top with champagne brut

Directions:

Shake the first three ingredients with ice and strain into chilled glass. Top with champagne. Garnish using lemon zest twist.

Fog Chopper

Preparation time: 10 minutes

Servings: 2

Ingredients:

15 milliliters almond (orgeat) syrup

15 milliliters amontillado sherry

15 milliliters lemon juice

15 milliliters London dry gin

22 milliliters Cognac V.S.O.P.

45 milliliters light white rum

45 milliliters orange juice

Directions:

Shake the first six ingredients with ice and strain into ice-filled glass. Float sherry on top of the drink. Garnish using an orange wedge.

Flash Tornado

Preparation time: 10 minutes

Servings: 2

Ingredients:

30 milliliters dry vermouth

30 milliliters London dry gin

30 milliliters orange juice

3 dashes peach bitters

Directions:

Shake ingredients with ice and strain into chilled glass. Garnish using orange zest twist.

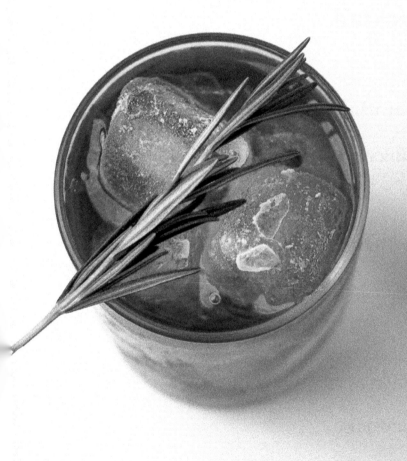

Whiskey Keto Cocktails

Tennessee Rye Brunswick cocktail

Preparation time: 10 minutes

Servings: 2

Ingredients:

2 parts of Jack Daniele's Tennessee rye

¾ claret red wine

½ simple syrup

¾ lemon juice

Orange slice

Cherry

Directions:

Combine lemon juice, simple syrup, Jack Daniele's Tennessee rye into a shaker with ice and shake it.

Strain into a glass over fresh ice

Make the wine float on top

Take the orange together with the cherry and use it to garnish

Serve while chilled

Apple Cider Punch

Preparation time: 10 minutes

Servings: 5

Ingredients:

4 to 6 cups apple cider

1 cup applejack or Calvados

Pinch of ground cloves

1 cup Irish whiskey

Garnish: 1 red Delicious apple, halved and sliced thin, and 1 lime, sliced

1/4 cup fresh lime juice, strained

Directions:

Mix apple cider, lime juice, whiskey, and applejack in a punch bowl. Add in cloves and stir. Refrigerate for 1 hour. Fill in ice cubes or a block of ice. Use lime slices and apples to decorate the punch.

Cameron's Kick

Preparation time: 10 minutes

Servings: 1

Ingredients:

3/4 oz. Scotch whiskey

3/4 oz. Irish whiskey

1/2 tbsp. lemon juice

1/2 tbsp. orgeat syrup (or 2 dashes of orange bitters)

3 or 4 ice cubes

Directions:

In a cocktail shaker, mix all ingredients and shake forcefully. Transfer into a cocktail glass through a strainer.

Espresso old fashioned

Preparation time: 10 minutes

Servings: 2

Ingredients:

60ml redemption rye whiskey

Lemon twist

60ml espresso or cold-brew coffee

7.5ml simple syrup

1 dash Peychaud's bitters

1 dash Absinthe

Directions:

Place a dash of absinthe in a glass

Pour rye whiskey, espresso, simple syrup into a glass and mix with ice

Prepare a glass with an ice cube and strain over it.

Squeeze oil from a lemon twist and prepare it as garnish.

Serve

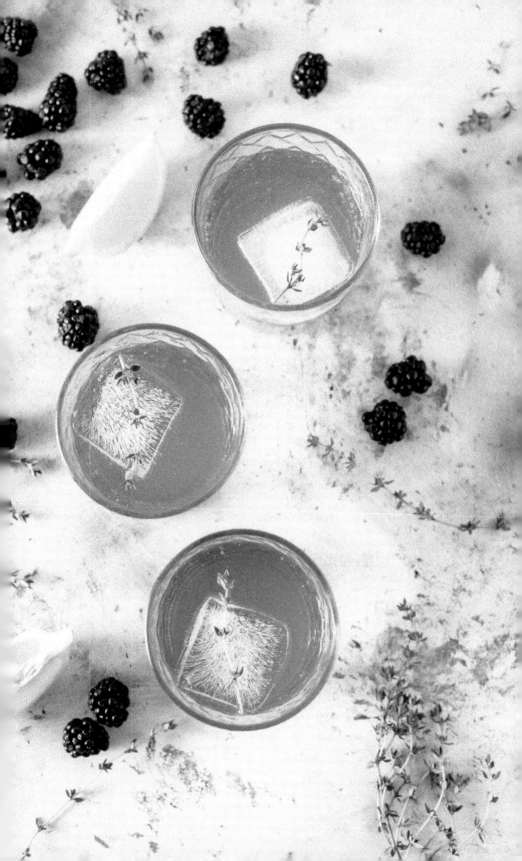

Tequila Cocktails

Galentine Cocktail

Preparation time: 5 minutes

Servings: 3

Ingredients:

1 cup pink lemonade

¼ cup lemon-lime soda

¼ cup fresh lemon juice

½ cup triple sec

1 cup tequila

Lemon slices, garnish

Ice

Directions:

Stir together pink lemonade, lemon-lime soda, lemon juice, triple sec, and tequila in a large pitcher with ice.

Pour into glasses and garnish with lemon slices.

Tequila Cup

Preparation time: 10 minutes

Servings: 2

Ingredients:

½ ounce orange curaçao

1 strawberry, hulled

1½ ounces 1800 Silver tequila

3 cucumber half-wheels

3 mint leaves

3 ounces Fresh Sour

7-Up, as required

Optional fruit: peach, apple, pear, tangerine, berries, etc.

Directions:

Mix all of the ingredients in a cocktail shaker with ice.

Shake casually and pour contents into a big glass.

Top with a splash of 7-Up.

Serve with a straw.

Agave Punch

Preparation time: 10 minutes

Servings: 2

Ingredients:

1 cup water

1 ounce triple sec

2 ounces pure agave reposado tequila

6 ounces frozen limeade concentrate

Lime half-wheels, for decoration (not necessary)

Directions:

Mix all of the ingredients apart from the lime half-wheel in a blender with four to 5 ice cubes.

Blend until the desired smoothness is achieved.

The mixture should not be too thick.

Pour into little cups and decorate each with a lime half-wheel.

Red Pepper Sangrita

Preparation time: 10 minutes

Servings: 1

Ingredients:

1½ ounces pure agave silver tequila

2½ ounces Pepper Mix (see below)

Whole red chili pepper, for decoration

Directions:

Mix the Pepper Mix and tequila in a cocktail shaker with ice.

Stir thoroughly (about ten seconds), strain into a chilled martini glass, and decorate with the red chili pepper.

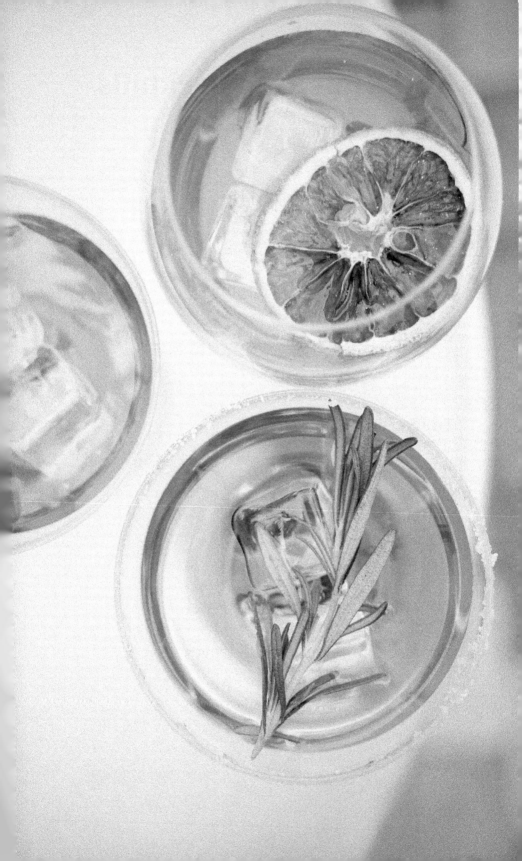

Rum Keto Cocktails

Blueberry Mojito

Preparation time: 10 minutes

Servings: 2

Ingredients:

3 lemons, chopped

350 ml (11.8 oz.) white rum

100 g (3.4 oz.) blueberries

600 ml (20.2 oz.) sparkling water

2 bruised mint sprigs, with leaves

2 tbsp granulated sugar

Directions:

In a jar, muddle the lemons, blueberries, and sugar together to get a syrup-like mixture.

Add the mint leaves and some ice cubes to the jar.

Pour the water and the rum, and stir everything together.

Strawberry Mojito

Preparation time: 10 minutes

Servings: 2

Ingredients:

350 ml (11.8oz.) white rum

2 limes, chopped

600 ml (20.3 oz.) sparkling water

Black pepper

2 tbsp granulated sugar

Ice cubes

2 mint sprigs, with leaves

10 strawberries

Directions:

In a jug, mix the strawberries, sugar, and limes until you get a creamy texture.

Bruise some mint leaves and add to the strawberry mixture, along with some black pepper.

Stir in the sparkling water and the rum.

Serve with ice cubes.

Sangrum

Preparation time: 10 minutes

Servings: 2

Ingredients:

½ cup chopped pineapple

½ cup light rum

1 apple, cored and cut

1 bottle of red wine

1 lemon, cut into wheels

1 liter 7-Up

1 pint strawberries, hulled and cut

12 whole cloves

2 limes, cut into wheels

2 oranges, cut into wedges

Directions:

Stick the cloves in the orange wedges or apple slices.

Mix the orange wedges and apple slices with all of the rest of the ingredients except the 7-Up in a big ceramic or glass container and stir thoroughly.

Cover and place in your fridge for a minimum of 4 hours (preferably overnight).

Just before you serve, put in the 7-Up.

Serve over ice.

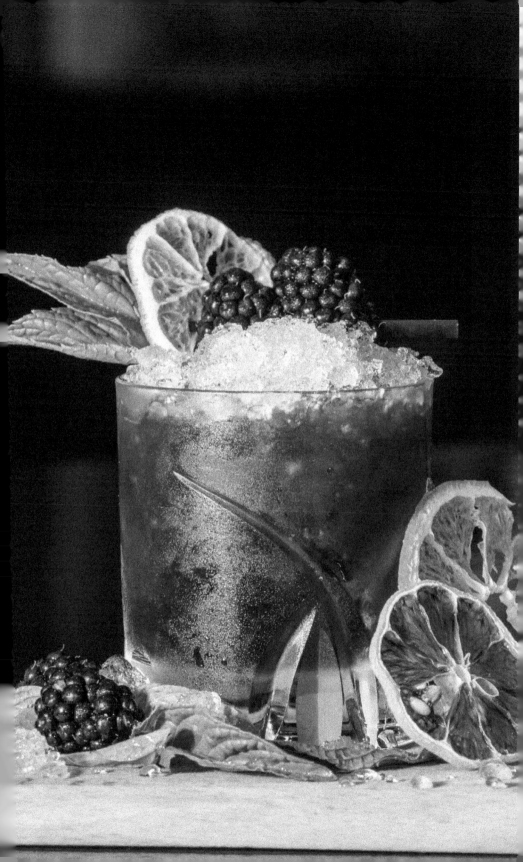

Vodka Keto Cocktails

Woo Woo

Preparation time: 10 minutes

Servings: 2

Ingredients:

100 ml (3.4 oz.) cranberry juice

50 ml (1.7 oz.) vodka

The juice of ½ lemon

24 ml (0.8 oz.) peach schnapps

Ice cubes

Lime wedges

Directions:

Put all the liquid ingredients, the lime juice, and some ice into your cocktail shaker, and shake well.

Strain the cocktail into a tumbler, and add additional ice.

Garnish with lime wedges before serving.

Sex on The Beach

Preparation time: 10 minutes

Servings: 2

Ingredients:

50 ml (1.7 oz.) vodka

50 ml (1.7 oz.) cranberry juice

25 ml (0.85 oz.) peach schnapps

The juice of 2 oranges

Glacé cherries to garnish

Ice cubes

Orange slices, to garnish

Directions:

Fill the glasses with ice cubes.

Pour the fruit juices, vodka, and peach schnapps into a large jug. Stir everything together.

Pour the mixture into the two glasses and stir once again.

Garnish with the cherries and additional orange slices before serving.

Bloody Mary

Preparation time: 10 minutes

Servings: 2

Ingredients:

200 ml (6.7 oz.) tomato juice

1 tsp sherry vinegar

50 ml (1.7 oz.) vodka

Ice cubes

2 tbsp amontillado sherry

A pinch of salt

Tabasco, to taste

Worcestershire sauce, to taste

Lemon juice

Celery sticks, to garnish

Lemon wedges, to garnish

Pepper, to serve (optional)

Directions:

Pour the vodka, tomato juice, sherry vinegar, and amontillado into a tall glass along with some ice cubes.

Season with Tabasco, celery salt, and Worcestershire sauce. Add lemon juice to taste.

Serve with lemon wedges, celery sticks, and freshly ground black (optional).

Long Island Iced Tea

Preparation time: 10 minutes

Servings: 2

Ingredients:

50 ml (1.7 oz.) London dry gin

50 ml (1.7 oz.) vanilla vodka

50 ml (1.7 oz.) tequila

50 ml (1.7 oz.) triple sec

50 ml (1.7 oz.) rum

50 ml (1.7 oz.) fresh lime juice

500 ml (17 oz.) cola

2 limes, cut into wedges

Ice cubes

Directions:

Pour all the spirits and liqueur into a large jug. Add lime juice.

Fill ½ of the jug with ice cubes and stir well.

Fill the jug with cola and stir once again.

Add the lime wedges and serve the cocktail into 4 tall glasses with additional ice cubes.

Espresso Martini

Preparation time: 10 minutes

Servings: 2

Ingredients:

100 ml (3.4 oz.) vodka

100 g (3.4 oz.) golden caster syrup

50 ml (1.7 oz.) coffee liqueur

50 ml (1.7 oz.) freshly brewed espresso

A few coffee beans, to garnish

Directions:

Bring the caster sugar to boil in 50 ml (1.7 oz.) of water. Allow the mixture to cool, stirring frequently until you obtain the right consistency for your sugar syrup.

Pour 1 tbsp of this sugar into a cocktail shaker with all the other ingredients.

Shake well and serve into 2 refrigerated martini glasses.

Garnish with additional coffee beans.

Caipiroska

Preparation time: 5 minutes

Servings: 2

Ingredients:

2 oz. vodka

¾ oz. sugar syrup

Ice

Lime

Directions:

Place 2 lime wedges into a rocks glass and muddle

Fill a rocks glass to the top with ice

Pour in ¾ oz. of sugar syrup and 2 oz. of vodka

Stir gently

Top up with crushed ice

Garnish with lemon slices

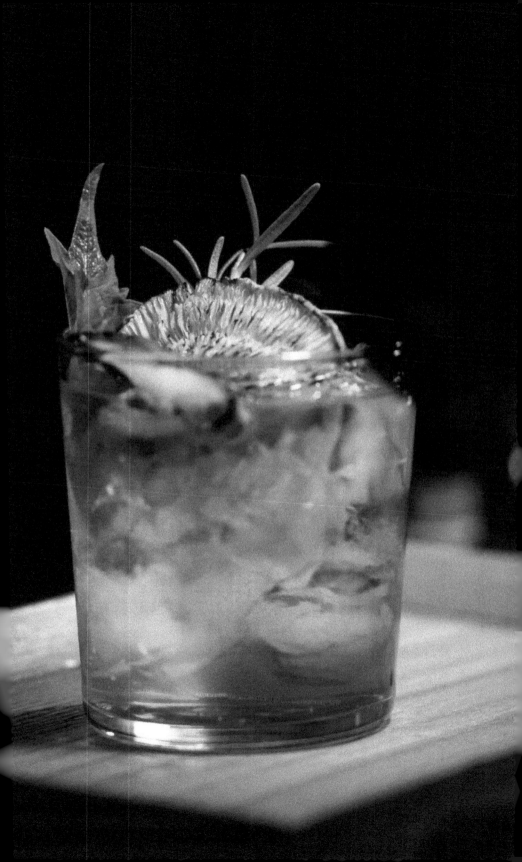

Keto Liqueurs

Coffee liqueur

Preparation time: 60 minutes

Servings: 3

Ingredients:

15.8oz. of mocha coffee or espresso

15.8oz. of sugar

Alcohol

Directions:

To prepare the Coffee Liqueur, start by preparing the coffee with the mocha (or if you prefer with the coffee machine,) which you will pour into a pan with high edges. Add the sugar and light the very low heat to melt it.

To facilitate the operation, you can mix with a spatula or with a wooden spoon. When the sugar is completely dissolved, pour the mixture into a small bowl to cool.

When it is well cooled, add the alcohol and mix it carefully with the other ingredients.

Finally, distribute Coffee Liqueur in new or well-washed glass bottles, perfectly clean and dried (once washed, it is advisable to dry them upside down on a clean towel). Screw the cap on and close the bottles tightly so that no air enters. Let Coffee Liqueur rest in the bottles for at least 2 weeks before consuming it.

Cherry liqueur

Preparation time: 2 days

Servings: 3

Ingredients:

14.1oz. of pitted cherries

14.1oz. of pure alcohol (~95°)

18.3oz. of water

3.3oz. of sugar

Directions:

To prepare Cherry Liqueur, first, wash and dry the cherries. Add the cherries to a glass jar, add the alcohol, close with the lid and leave to macerate at room temperature for a week.

After the maceration time, take the jar again, filter the mixture through a strainer and collect the infusion in a container. Pour sugar into a saucepan.

Add the water and heat the syrup over medium heat for 15 minutes. Let the syrup cool slightly, then add it to the infusion.

Mix in the Liqueur obtained, pour it into a jar with an airtight seal, and let it rest for 3 weeks at room temperature. After this time, your Cherry Liqueur will be ready: pour it in a bottle and keep it at room temperature, if it is not too hot, or place it in the refrigerator.

Tips:

Cherry Liqueur can be kept for 90 days in the refrigerator or at room temperature if it is not too hot. Once opened, it is preferable to keep it in the refrigerator.

If you like an extra aromatic touch, add vanilla seeds, cinnamon sticks, or orange zest to your liqueur.

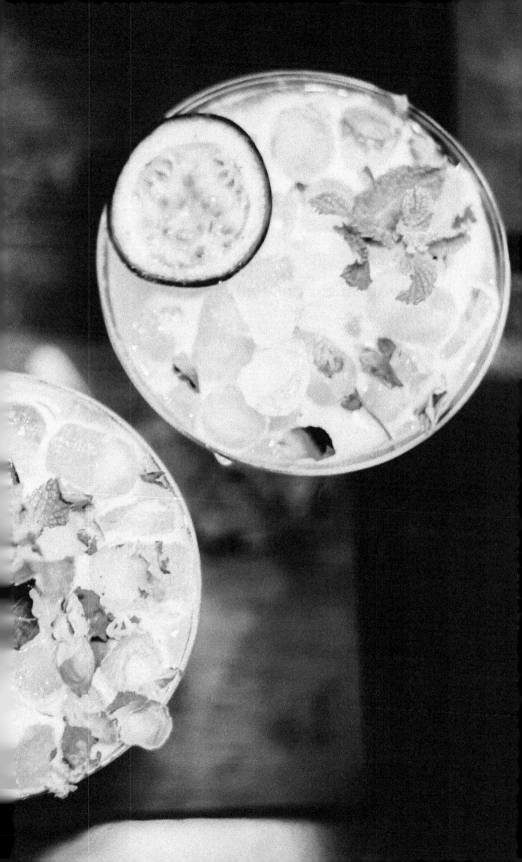

Keto Mocktails

Mint Julep Mocktail

Preparation time: 60 minutes

Servings: 3

Ingredients:

¼ cup water (filtered)

¼ cup of sugar, white

1 tbsp. of mint leaves (fresh, chopped)

2 cups of ice (crushed)

½ cup of lemonade (ready-made)

For Garnishing:

Fresh sprigs of mint

Directions:

Combine filtered water, white sugar, and 1 tbsp. chopped mint leaves. Stir, bring to boil.

Cook mixture until sugar is dissolved. Remove from heat. Set aside for cooling.

After an hour or so, strain the mint leaves out.

Fill two cups with crushed ice. Add half lemonade in each cup. Top with a splash of sugar syrup.

Garnish cups with straw and sprig of mint. Serve.

Arnold Palmer

Preparation time: 5 minutes

Servings: 3

Ingredients:

2 parts of iced tea for each

1 part of lemonade for each

For garnishing:

slices of lemon

Directions:

Pour iced tea and lemonade into two ice-filled tall glasses.

Stir thoroughly.

Garnish with lemon slices. Serve.

Raspberry-Cranberry Twist

Preparation time: 10 minutes

Servings: 3

Ingredients:

1 x 12 fluid oz. bottle or can of carbonated beverage (lemon-lime flavor)

12 fluid oz. of cranberry-raspberry juice

Directions:

Mix the lemon-lime soda with cranberry-raspberry juice. Pour it over ice. Serve.

Sweet Virgin Sunrise

Preparation time: 5 minutes

Servings: 3

Ingredients:

4 fluid oz. of orange juice (fresh-squeezed if possible)

Ice

½ fluid oz. of grenadine

Orange slice for garnishing

Directions:

Pour ice into a highball glass and add the orange juice.

Pour grenadine slowly over juice.

Use an orange slice to garnish and serve.

Chicha Morada

Preparation time: 5hour

Servings: 3

Ingredients:

1 (3½ pound) fresh pineapple

2 Granny Smith apples (cored)

1 (16 ounce) bag dried purple corn

2 (2") sticks of cinnamon

½ tsp whole cloves

¾ cup packed light brown sugar

7 pints water

½ cup + 2 tbsp freshly squeezed lemon juice

½ cup + 2 tbsp freshly squeezed lime juice

1 tsp kosher salt

Wheels of fresh lime (to garnish)

Ice (to serve)

Directions:

Trim, peel, and core the pineapple. Set the peel and core to one side.

Dice ¼ of the diced pineapple (approximately 1 cup) and set the remaining aside for alternative use.

Cut one of the cored apples into quarters.

In a large size pan, combine the pineapple peel, pineapple core, and apple with the corn, cinnamon stick, cloves, brown sugar, and 7 pints of water).

Cover the pan with a lid and over moderate-high heat, bring to boil.

Remove the lid, and turn the heat down to moderate. Simmer the corn until it softens and the liquid slightly reduces, for approximately 60 minutes.

With a slotted spoon, remove any solids and discard them.

Pour the liquid through a strainer into a large size heat-safe bowl and allow it to stand for 45 minutes, or until it no longer steams.

Whisk in the fresh lemon juice followed by the lime juice and salt, and transfer to the fridge for 2 hours, until cold.

Peel the remaining apple and dice.

Add the diced apple and diced pineapple to a punch bowl or large pitcher.

Pour the Chicha Morada over the fruit, garnish with wheels of fresh lime, and serve with ice.

Mint watermelon

Preparation time: 10 minutes

Servings: 4

Ingredients:

1/2 cup cold-pressed watermelon juice

1 tablespoon. freshly squeezed lime

2 mint leaves

fresh mint for garnish

lime zest for garnish

Directions:

Pour all the ingredients into a shaker with a handful of ice. Shake for 30 seconds to 1 minute.

Garnish with fresh mint and lime zest.

Serve on ice.

Peach and rosemary iced tea

Preparation time: 10 minutes

Servings: 4

Ingredients:

1 dl of water

75 g of sugar

200 g of diced peaches

For the mocktail:

¾ of a liter of water

1 Earl Gray Everton teabag

3 sprigs of rosemary

½ lemon

½ peach in wedges

Directions:

Boil the water with the sugar in a saucepan. Add the peaches and cook for about 10 minutes. Now, remove from the heat and let the syrup flavor for about an hour.

Meanwhile, boil the tea water and let our Earl Gray with rosemary infuse for about 15 minutes. Remove the sachets and the rosemary and add the peach syrup and the juice of ½ lemon. Let it cool and put everything in the refrigerator for about 1 hour. Serve it to your guests with peach wedges, rosemary, and ice cubes.

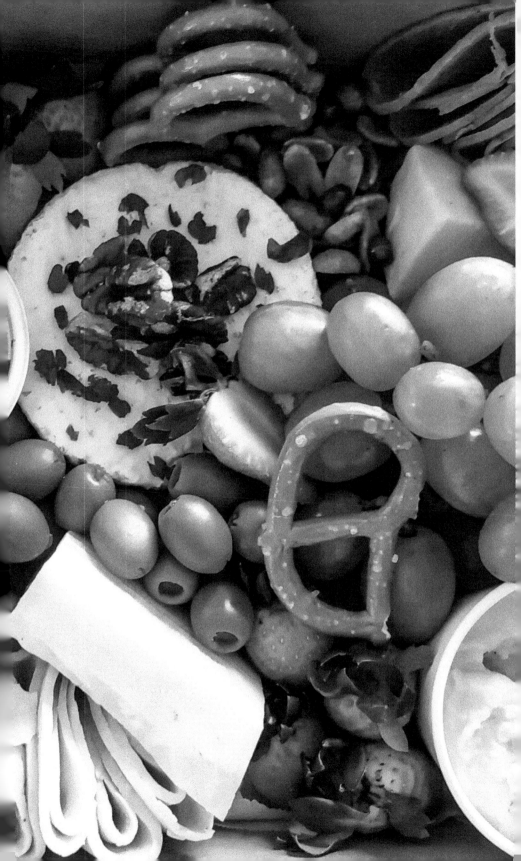

Keto Snacks for Happy Hour

Mushroom and Asparagus Frittata

Preparation time: 10 minutes

Cooking Time: 45 minutes

Servings: 8

Ingredients:

8 large eggs

1/2 cup of ricotta cheese

2 tbsps. of lemon juice

1/2 tsp. of salt

1/4 tsp. of pepper

1 tbsp. of olive oil

8 ounces of asparagus spears

1 onion (sliced)

1/3 cup of sweet green pepper

3/4 cup of Portobello mushrooms (sliced)

Directions:

Preheat your oven at one hundred and fifty degrees Celsius. Combine ricotta cheese, eggs, pepper, lemon juice, and salt in a bowl. Heat oil in an iron skillet. Add onion, asparagus, mushrooms, and red pepper. Cook for eight minutes. Remove the asparagus from the skillet.

Cut the spears of asparagus into pieces of two-inch. Return the spears to the skillet. Add the mixture of eggs. Bake in the oven for twenty minutes. Let the frittata sit for five minutes.

Cut the frittata into wedges. Serve warm.

Nutrition: calories 200, fat 8, fiber 4, carbs 8, protein 3

Sausage Balls

Preparation time: 10 minutes

Cooking Time: 45 minutes

Servings: 6

Ingredients:

1 pound of spicy pork sausage (ground)

8 ounces of cream cheese

1/2 cup of cheddar cheese (shredded)

1/3 cup of parmesan cheese (shredded)

1 tbsp. of Dijon mustard

1/2 tsp. of garlic powder

1/4 tsp. of salt

Directions:

Preheat your oven at one hundred and seventy degrees Celsius. Use parchment paper for lining a baking sheet. Combine cream cheese, sausage, parmesan cheese, cheddar cheese, garlic powder, mustard, and salt in a mixing bowl. Mix well.

Take one tbsp. of the mixture. Roll it into a ball. Repeat for the remaining mixture. Arrange the prepared balls on the lined baking tray. Bake for thirty minutes.

Serve hot.

Nutrition: calories 110, fat 10, fiber 1, carbs 3, protein 6

Ranch Cauliflower Crackers

Preparation time: 10 minutes

Cooking Time: 30 minutes

Servings: 6

Ingredients:

12 ounces of cauliflower rice

Cheesecloth

1 large egg

1 tbsp. of ranch salad dressing mix (dry)

1/8 tsp. of cayenne pepper

1 cup of parmesan cheese (shredded)

Directions:

Add the cauliflower rice to a large bowl. Microwave for four minutes covered. Transfer the cauliflower rice to a strainer lined with cheesecloth. Squeeze out excess moisture. Preheat the oven to two hundred degrees Celsius. Use parchment paper for lining a baking tray.

Combine egg, cauliflower rice, ranch mix, and pepper in a bowl. Add the cheese. Mix well. Take two tbsps. Of the mixture and add them to the baking tray. Flatten with your hands. The thinner you can make the mixture; the crispier will be the crackers.

Bake for ten minutes. Flip the crackers. Bake for ten minutes. Serve warm.

Nutrition: calories 110, fat 10, fiber 1, carbs 3, protein 6

Pork Belly Cracklings

Preparation time: 10 minutes

Cooking Time: 80 minutes

Servings: 6

Ingredients:

3 pounds of pork belly (with skin)

2 cups of water

4 tbsps. of Cajun seasoning

Directions:

Keep the pork belly in the refrigerator for forty minutes. Cut the pork into cubes of a three-fourth inch. Fill a cast-iron pot with one-fourth portion of water. Add one tsp. of Cajun seasoning. Boil the water.

Add the cubes of pork belly. Cook for twenty minutes. Cover the pot once fat begins to pop and sizzle. Cook for fifteen minutes. Drain the pork cracklings.

Sprinkle remaining seasoning from the top. Serve immediately.

Nutrition: calories 383, fat 14, fiber 4, carbs 3, protein 8

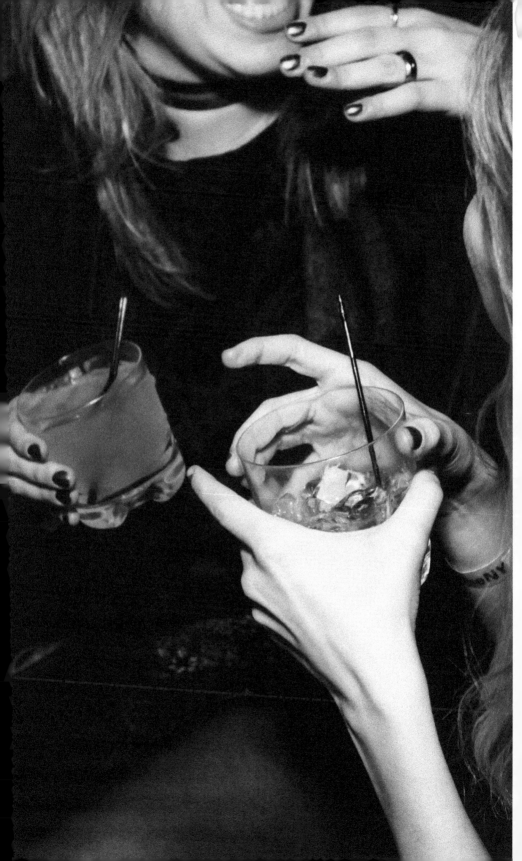

Conclusion

This book will help you kickstart your fitness journey and ultimately support you in reaching your ideal body weight. Start by understanding how Keto Cocktail works and choose a cocktail that suits your needs. Find out which drinks you can drink and which ones you should avoid, calculate your macros, plan your meals and make a list of food items you need to buy. To increase results, incorporate some form of exercise every day. It could be a 30 minute walk or a high intensity training session. Whatever you do never give up live your keto life!

Lightning Source UK Ltd.
Milton Keynes UK
UKHW020637030621
384863UK00011B/1258